WS 110 BER

Library Alliance

D0026457

Developing [
Health Servi
Children and Adolescents
wi   ities

D0538185

20830941
BER.

A T

DATE DUE			

Developing Mental Health Services for Children and Adolescents with Learning Disabilities

A Toolkit for Clinicians

Edited by Dr Sarah Bernard
& Professor Jeremy Turk

RCPsych Publications
in collaboration with the National CAMHS Support Service

© The Royal College of Psychiatrists 2009

RCPsych Publications is an imprint of the Royal College of Psychiatrists,
17 Belgrave Square, London SW1X 8PG
http://www.rcpsych.ac.uk

All rights reserved. No part of this book may be reprinted or reproduced or utilised in any form or by any electronic, mechanical, or other means, now known or hereafter invented, including photocopying and recording, or in any information storage or retrieval system, without permission in writing from the publishers.

British Library Cataloguing-in-Publication Data.
A catalogue record for this book is available from the British Library.
ISBN 978-1-904671-61-9

Distributed in North America by Balogh International Inc.

The views presented in this book do not necessarily reflect those of the Royal College of Psychiatrists, and the publishers are not responsible for any error of omission or fact.

The Royal College of Psychiatrists is a charity registered in England and Wales (228636) and in Scotland (SC038369).

Printed UK by Bell & Bain Limited, Glasgow.

Contents

Contributors

Tamsin Arnold, DClinPsy, Consultant Clinical Psychologist, The Children with Disabilities Behaviour and Family Support Team, Royal Borough of Kensington and Chelsea/Central and North West London NHS Foundation Trust, London

Sarah H. Bernard, MD FRCPsych DRCOG, Consultant Psychiatrist, Child and Adolescent Learning Disability, South London and Maudsley NHS Foundation Trust, London

Vivien Cooper, Parent and Trustee of the Challenging Behaviour Foundation

Alison Dunkerley, MB ChB MRCPsych, Consultant Learning Disability Child Psychiatrist, 5 Boroughs Partnership NHS Trust, St Helens, Lancashire

Dido Green, PhD MSc DipCOT, Clinical Expert Occupational Therapist, Paediatric Neurosciences, Guy's Hospital, London

Felicity Hepper, MRCPsych, Consultant Child and Adolescent Psychiatrist, Brent Child and Adolescent Mental Health Service, Central and North West London NHS Foundation Trust, London

Jen Jenkin, MRCSLT, Principal Speech and Language Therapist, Northumberland, Tyne and Wear NHS Trust

Tony O'Sullivan, FRCP FRCPCH DCH, Consultant Paediatrician and Clinical Director, Kaleidoscope Lewisham Centre for Children and Young People, Lewisham Primary Care Trust

David Smith, MSc BSc(Hons) RMN RNMH, Clinical Nurse Specialist, Wandsworth Child and Adolescent Mental Health Learning Disability Service, South West London and St George's Mental Health NHS Trust

Helen Stringer, PhD MRCSLT, Director of Clinical Education/Speech and Language Therapist, School of Education, Communication and Language Sciences, Newcastle University

Harry Tuck, Social Worker, Project Manager, Lambeth Children and Young People's Service

Jeremy Turk, MD BSc(Hons) FRCPsych FRCPCH DCH, Professor of Developmental Psychiatry, St George's, University of London, and Consultant Child and Adolescent Psychiatrist, South West London & St George's Mental Health NHS Trust

Foreword

We are delighted to welcome you to this practical toolkit, which, in its brief and easy-to-read format, outlines the key principles to consider when working with children and young people with a learning disability who have a mental health problem.

The National Service Framework for Children is now in its fifth year and the Public Service Agreement 12 (2007), as part of the Comprehensive Spending Review, set out the government's vision for improving the physical, mental and emotional health of all children and re-emphasised the needs of children and young people with a learning disability. While we recognise that much progress has already been made in this field, we also know there is still a need to embed quality commissioning and provider services for all children and young people and in particular for those who have learning disabilities, in order that they have access to truly comprehensive child and adolescent mental health services which meet all their needs.

This toolkit is written by clinicians for clinicians. It emphasises the clinical, practical and theoretical perspectives which will help build a more capable workforce and deliver services that improve the life chances of this group of children.

It is a further contribution to the range of toolkits and resources which champion the needs of this group of children, such as the 'Do Once and Share' project and its care pathway, and which have been helpful in developing our thinking about what kind of support and developments ensure that appropriate levels of service are commissioned and provided. This toolkit adds to that body of work and extends it.

This toolkit is an *aide-mémoire* for mental health professionals when starting out in clinical practice. It aims to support their work with children and young people with learning disabilities and covers the topic areas which are relevant to most cases. No handbook, however, can be exhaustive, so the reader will find references for further reading at the end of each chapter. Skills build over time as experience expands, and we hope that this publication will be a useful contribution to professional development for all staff working with this group of young people.

Respected clinicians and practitioners voluntarily contributed their experience to each of the chapters. Our thanks go to them. Our particular thanks go to the clinical editors, Dr Sarah Bernard and Professor Jeremy Turk, who edited the contributors' drafts and organised the material into a coherent whole. It is typical of their unstinting commitment to improving the lives of this group of children and young people that they never turn down an opportunity to make a difference!

Dawn Rees
National CAMHS Strategic Relationships and Programme Manager.
National CAMHS Support Service
www.cypf.csip.org.uk

Preface

It is widely recognised that although young people with learning disability are at an increased risk of mental health or behavioural problems, there is a serious lack of appropriate mental health provision to meet these needs. The National Service Framework for Children states clearly that services should be available to all. Other documentation has also emphasised this need but, unfortunately, the provision of child and adolescent mental health services (CAMHS) for this group of young people remains inadequate.

This toolkit, we hope, will, along with other recent publications, help CAMHS clinicians to feel more confident in assessing and managing the basic mental health needs of these children and young people in a multidisciplinary manner. We hope that it will help abolish the discriminatory 'IQ lottery' of access to CAMHS provision for children with learning disability.

The term 'learning disability' is generally used throughout this text. Although 'intellectual disability' is now more commonly used internationally and in the scientific literature, 'learning disability' is more widespread within the context of the UK National Health Service and so is preferred here.

We would like to thank all the people who have contributed to this publication. Particular thanks go to Mary Killick, CAMHS Regional Development Worker, Care Services Improvement Partnership, for her support, enthusiasm and encouragement.

Sarah H. Bernard
Jeremy Turk

Abbreviations

ADHD	attention-deficit hyperactivity disorder
CAMHS	child and adolescent mental health service
SLT	speech and language therapy
SSRI	selective serotonin reuptake inhibitor

CHAPTER 1

Epidemiological overview

Children and adolescents with developmental disabilities are at a greater risk of developing mental health or behavioural problems than are their non-disabled peers. This fact is supported by several epidemiological studies:

- Rutter *et al* (1970) studied 10- to 12-year-old children on the Isle of Wight and found that emotional and behavioural disorders were much commoner in children with learning disabilities.
- Corbett (1979) showed in a study of children with severe learning disability aged 0–15 years in south-east London that 47% of the sample had some form of psychiatric disorder.
- Gillberg *et al* (1986), in a study of 13- to 17-year-olds in Sweden, demonstrated increased rates of autism, language and social impairment and psychosis in those with an IQ of less than 50.
- Emerson & Hatton (2007) studied 641 children with learning disabilities and found higher rates of social disadvantage and an increased risk of all psychiatric disorders.

It is also recognised that these children are less likely to access appropriate mental health services. Even when they do, they are less likely to have their psychiatric and developmental needs recognised, understood and addressed in an evidence-based and optimally therapeutic fashion. Child and adolescent mental health services (CAMHS) are, in general, lacking in the expertise and resources required to provide comprehensive assessments and ongoing management for those with developmental disabilities. This affects the child's mental health, and educational and social needs. Additionally, there is a negative impact on family life, with an increased likelihood of sibling and parental emotional distress, family breakdown and expensive residential placements. Research findings are consistent with a good third of children and young people with learning disability experiencing mental health problems, compared with 11% of those who have only a physical disability or chronic illness, and 8% of children and young people in the general population. In a single London borough, where the population is approximately 250 000, 20% (approximately 50 000) of these being children and young people, one should expect 2–3% (approximately 1500) to have a learning disability, with approximately 250 of these having an IQ of less than 50. A good third of those with mild learning disability will have mental health problems that are diagnosable and for which help can be offered; untreated, however, these problems lead inevitably to significantly impaired quality of life and underachievement. This amounts to approximately 420 individuals. A good half of those with moderate-to-profound learning disability will have mental health problems that are both diagnosable and for which help is available, amounting to a further 125 individuals. Thus, at any time, there are approximately 550 children and young people in just one London borough who have learning disability meriting mental health evaluation and input.

Individuals with learning disability are also acknowledged as being at increased risk of autistic-spectrum disorders and attention-deficit hyperactivity disorder (ADHD). Epidemiological data suggest that in a similar population to that above there should be approximately 250 children with autistic-spectrum disorders and 2000 children and young people with ADHD, and many from both these groups will have a learning disability as well. This gives some idea of the magnitude and pressing nature of these public health issues.

Mental health disorders commonly encountered in children and adolescents with learning disability

Children and adolescents with learning disability are likely to encounter the same range of psychiatric disorders as their non-learning disabled peers, although certain disorders are more common than others.

Standardised diagnostic criteria should be considered with the understanding that symptoms and phenomena should be interpreted in the light of the child's level of cognitive functioning and understanding. In addition, physical and sensory disabilities will influence the presentation of a psychiatric disorder, as will associated social and communication difficulties.

The account that follows is by no means comprehensive and readers should refer to the texts listed at the end of this chapter to gain further information about specific disorders.

Autism and autistic-spectrum disorders

These disorders have the following characteristics:

- they are pervasive
- they usually manifest before the child is aged 3 years
- there is abnormal functioning in all three areas of social interaction, communication and behaviour (which is restrictive and repetitive).

In children with severe learning disability, the level of cognitive functioning should be considered when considering the triad of autistic symptoms. Certain behaviours that appear autistic may, in fact, be appropriate for the child's cognitive level. Conversely, it is quite possible, and is often the case, that a child's level and nature of social and communicatory functioning are sufficiently out of keeping with the child's general cognitive ability that they merit a diagnosis of autism in addition to learning disability.

The management of children with autism involves combined developmental, behavioural and educational approaches. Medication sometimes has a role but is not a first-line option and should always be used in conjunction with behavioural and other interventions.

Hyperactivity and attention-deficit hyperactivity disorder

Attention-deficit hyperactivity disorder (ADHD) has the following key characteristics:

- early onset – usually within the first 5 years of life
- overactive, poorly modulated behaviour with marked inattention and overactivity
- pervasiveness.

Associated abnormalities include restlessness, fidgetiness, impulsivity, distractibility, breaching of rules, social disinhibition and cognitive impairments.

ADHD is often under-diagnosed in children with developmental disabilities, because the child's lack of attention can be interpreted as being due to the underlying cognitive impairment rather than an associated attentional disorder.

The management of children with ADHD includes a trial of psychostimulant medication, behavioural approaches to maximise attentional and associated skills, and consideration of the educational and social environments.

Depression

The clinical manifestations of depression include:

- low mood
- loss of interest in daily activities
- loss of energy
- tearfulness
- poor concentration and memory
- biological features, including disturbed sleep, poor appetite and diurnal mood variation
- low self-esteem and negative view of the future

- distress
- self-injury.

Distress can be mistaken for depression. Conversely, treatable depression is often missed because behavioural change is explained away as being part of the general presentation of the individual's learning disability (this is termed 'diagnostic overshadowing') or is labelled as 'challenging behaviour'.

In children and adolescents who are non-verbal, diagnosis relies largely on the biological and somatic features of depression, often as reported by others.

As in children without developmental disabilities, depression can resolve spontaneously, but the risk of relapse must be considered. Cognitive–behavioural therapies can be helpful in initial episodes of mild to moderate depression, but if unsuccessful, a cautious trial of medication should be considered, usually a selective serotonin reuptake inhibitor (SSRI) in combination with cognitive–behavioural work.

Psychosis – including schizophrenia and bipolar disorder

The clinical manifestations of psychosis include:

- thought disorder
- hallucinations
- delusions
- catatonic behaviours
- negative features, including apathy, blunting of affect and social withdrawal
- changes in behaviour.

In schizophrenia, the above symptoms are incongruent with mood, while in bipolar affective disorder they are mood congruent. Distinguishing between the two types of psychotic disorder is often problematic in children and adolescents with moderate to profound learning disability and hence treatment often needs to be pragmatic and empirical.

A diagnosis of psychosis should be made only by experienced clinicians, as once the label had been given, it will have major implications for the child's educational placement, for access to respite services and for service provision in adulthood.

Antipsychotic medication must be supervised. The current treatments of choice are atypical neuroleptics such as risperidone, olanzepine, quetiapine and aripiprazole. In bipolar disorder, mood stabilisers have a role. Monitoring of lithium levels can pose difficulties. Thus sodium valproate or carbamazepine may, in certain instances, offer a safer alternative.

Tourette syndrome

The syndrome is characterised by:

4

- multiple motor tics
- one or more vocal tics often accompanied by explosive vocalisations
- onset in childhood or adolescence.

Support and psychoeducation for parents and teachers are important. Medication such as risperidone, sulpiride, pimozide or clonidine reduces tic frequency but benefits must be balanced against the risks of side-effects.

External stressors increase the frequency of tics. Hence cognitive–behavioural approaches focusing on monitoring of environmental triggers, problem-solving and stress management can be useful.

Challenging behaviour

This is not a diagnosis. It is a descriptive term for any behaviour that poses a challenge for the individual, carers or society. Emerson (2001) defines challenging behaviour as a set of 'behaviours of such an intensity, frequency or duration that the physical safety of the person or others is likely to be placed in serious jeopardy, or behaviour is likely to seriously limit or delay access to and use of ordinary community facilities'.

Any behavioural problem requires a comprehensive assessment in order to identify causative factors (antecedents); this assessment must include underlying physical or psychiatric disorders as well as possible reinforcing consequences of the behaviours.

Challenging behaviours include:

- self-injury
- aggression
- persistent spitting
- self-induced vomiting
- persistent masturbation/sexualized behaviours

Challenging behaviours are more common in individuals with learning disability and autism, their frequency and intensity increasing with the severity of these conditions.

Management involves the multidisciplinary team, the family, the school and social services. Behavioural psychotherapy is the first line of approach but cautious use of medication may be indicated. This should be tailored to individual need.

Self-injury

This behaviour:

- is relatively common in children and adolescents with severe learning disability and autism
- may serve a variety of functions, including attention-seeking, gaining solitude, demand avoidance, over- or under-stimulation, self-stimulation, emotional reaction to bereavement, abuse or neglect

- may be part of a post-traumatic stress disorder
- may be a presenting feature of a specific syndrome, such as Lesch–Nyhan syndrome, Smith–Magenis syndrome, Prader–Willi syndrome, fragile-X syndrome, Cornelia de Lange syndrome.

Always consider social factors such as deprivation, disadvantage, neglect and abuse as underlying contributors. A detailed functional assessment is crucial. In the absence of environmental triggers consider using electro-enchephalography (EEG) to aid diagnosis.

Management combines behavioural psychotherapy with medication such as SSRIs, atypical antipsychotics, anticonvulsants, or opioid antagonists. Medication should be tailored to individual needs and given only for as brief a period as possible, and then under highly specialist supervision.

References

Corbett, J. A. (1979) Psychiatric morbidity and mental retardation. In *Psychiatric Illness and Mental Handicap* (eds F. E. James & R. P. Snaith). Gaskell.

Emerson, E. (2001) *Challenging Behaviour: Analysis and Intervention in People with Severe Intellectual Disabilities.* Cambridge University Press.

Emerson, E. & Hatton, C. (2007) Contribution of socioeconomic position to health inequalities of British children and adolescents with intellectual disabilities. *American Journal of Mental Retardation*, **112**, 140–150.

Gillberg, C., Persson, U., Grufman, M., *et al* (1986) Psychiatric disorders in mildly and severely mentally retarded urban children and adolescents. Epidemiological aspects. *British Journal of Psychiatry*, **149**, 69–74.

Rutter, M., Graham, P. & Yule, W. (1970) *A Neuropsychiatric Study in Childhood* (Clinics in Developmental Medicine Nos 35/36). Heinemann.

CHAPTER 2

Multidisciplinary mental health assessment

The aim of a multidisciplinary assessment is to undertake comprehensive and detailed evaluation of the individual from a wide range of biological, psychological, educational, developmental and social perspectives in order to achieve:

- a succinct yet informative formulation
- a set of differential diagnoses (or alternative explanations) for the nature of the presenting challenges
- a set of factors contributing to their likelihood (predisposing), occurrence (precipitating) and persistence (perpetuating)
- a profile of useful, cost-effective and evidence-based biopsychosocial interventions and supports likely to minimise the presenting challenges while maximising achievement of potential and quality of life for the individual and family.

How do mental health problems present in children with learning disability?

Mental health problems present in children with learning disability in just the same way as in children with more average intellectual functioning. The mental health worker, though, needs to beware of 'diagnostic overshadowing' (see p. 4). The presenting features can include:

- social, communicatory, ritualistic and obsessional impairments
- overactivity, attentional deficits
- aggression
- self-injurious behaviour
- cyclical mood and behaviour changes.

Diagnosis can be complicated by:

- frequent communication difficulties
- having to adjust for mental age.

Contributors to psychological difficulties in children and young people with learning disability

These include:
- the severity of the learning disability
- the cause of the learning disability
- the presence of autistic-spectrum disorder
- social factors –
  - abuse and neglect
  - schooling issues
  - poverty
  - parental psychiatric disorder
  - transgenerational social disadvantage
  - bereavement
  - life events, daily hassles, post-traumatic stress disorder
  - migration
  - attachment disorders.

Conditions causing, or complicating, presenting challenges

These include:
- neurodevelopmental disabilities
  - learning disability
  - autistic-spectrum disorders
  - attention-deficit disorders
- neuropsychiatric disorders
  - obsessive–compulsive disorder
  - cyclical mood disorder
  - depression
  - anxiety states
  - tics and Tourette syndrome
- psychosocial circumstances.

Types of diagnosis (and who usually makes it)

An aetiological diagnosis would be made by a paediatrician. Examples would include fragile-X syndrome, Down syndrome, foetal alcohol syndrome and congenital rubella.

A phenomenological diagnosis would be made by a mental health professional. Examples would include autism, Asperger syndrome, hyperactivity, ADHD, self–injury, 'challenging behaviour' and conduct disorder.

A descriptive of level of intellectual functioning would be made by an educationalist. An example would be 'moderate learning difficulties'.

A 'diagnosis' reflecting social factors would be made by social services, and could relate to inadequate housing or education, abuse, neglect. Similarly, a 'diagnosis' reflecting adverse interactions would be made by social services or a mental health professional (or both) and might relate to attachment disorder, family dysfunction or marital disharmony.

Presenting emotional and behavioural states

These presenting states may be:

- consistent with developmental level
- an understandable response to experiences (e.g. bereavement)
- the result of vulnerability produced by having learning disabilities
- indicative of a specific developmental delay (e.g. dyslexia, dyspraxia, attentional, social, communicatory)
- part of a 'general'' genetic predisposition
- specific to particular condition –
  - gaze aversion in fragile-X syndrome
  - hyperventilation and hand-wringing in Rett syndrome
  - overeating, obesity, impulsive tantrums and skin-picking in Prader–Willi syndrome
  - profound and intractable self-injury in Lesch–Nyhan syndrome.

Multifaceted evaluation

Evaluation should cover:

- psychiatric and developmental disorders
- characteristic behavioural profiles
- intellectual functioning –
  - level, profile, meaning
  - specific learning difficulties/developmental delays
- language and communication
- family and social
- educational
- other emotional problems
- other challenging behaviours.

Multi-faceted intervention

The intervention decided upon may need to include:

- education and information
- cognitive and behavioural psychotherapies
- family therapies
- speech and language therapy
- occupational therapy
- medication
- attention to social circumstances and social supports
- liaison and consultation
- counselling and support.

Classification of reasons for challenging behaviour:

Behaviour as part of a primary condition

Organic/biological causes

Such causes of challenging behaviour as part of a primary condition can be classified as:

- genetic (e.g. fragile-X or Down syndrome)
- toxic (e.g. foetal alcohol syndrome)
- infective (e.g. rubella)
- metabolic (e.g. phenylketonuria, hypothyroidism)
- malnutrition
- hypoxia
- physical brain trauma (e.g. from road traffic accident or child abuse).

Psychosocial causes

These include:

- profound deprivation, under-stimulation
- abuse and neglect.

Behaviour as a specific secondary consequence of the primary condition

Learning or other developmental disability may affect one or more further areas of development in such a way as to affect behaviour in a social setting:

- impaired social understanding
- impaired ability to relate socially
- impaired communication (e.g. misunderstandings, relative delay in response or failure to respond to verbal approaches from others, use of communicative behaviours which may be misinterpreted, such

as aggression 'without reason', literal use of language, repetitive expressive language).

Behaviour secondary to an unrelated physical condition

Limited communication skills can lead to pain and distress, for example, being expressed through challenging behaviour. The pain may be from, for example:

- earache
- gastro-oesophageal reflux ('heartburn")
- toothache
- arthritis
- intestinal blockage (constipation and faecal impaction)
- angina.

Behaviour as non-specific secondary consequence of impact of the primary condition

Behavioural and emotional disorders are commoner in children and young people with learning disability than in the age-matched general population.

Behaviour related to parenting and secondary impact of disability

The impact of the child's disability on the emotional and mental well-being of the child's carers and siblings needs to be considered.

Important competences

Learning disability specialists working on a CAMHS need to have:

- competence in the assessment of the level and profile of development (this can range from the basic, clinical–observational through the use of simple evaluation tools to comprehensive psychometric and speech and language therapy testing)
- working knowledge of key developmental milestones (motor, language, social, attentional, adaptive)
- the ability to recognise features suggestive of intellectual, social, linguistic and attentional developmental disorders which may present, or be associated, with emotional, behavioural and mental health difficulties
- an understanding of the relevance of laboratory and other biomedical investigations in the assessment process.

Referral pathways for initial assessment

Pre-school children with developmental and behavioural concerns are most likely to be referred to a child development service. School-age children with developmental, emotional and behavioural challenges are referred usually to the local CAMHS.

Following initial assessment some need referral from one team to another. A close working relationship is therefore essential between the child development team, the CAMHS, the local education authority and schools, local social services and local private and voluntary organisations. This is facilitated by a strong CAMHS presence in the multidisciplinary child development team.

Child development and warning signs of abnormal development

An individual's developmental progress varies enormously and is determined by a complex interplay between environmental factors (maternal health antenatally, *in utero* conditions, the birth process, economic and social conditions facing the family) and genetic factors.

A sound knowledge of typical child development is essential for recognition of common presentations when development is abnormal in one of the following ways:

- delayed rate of development (i.e. beyond accepted range of normal variation) in one or more developmental domains (e.g. echolalia still present by 3 years)
- absolute failure to develop skills (e.g. no 'canonical' babble – that is, repeated strings of expressive vocalisation of well-formed syllables, such as 'bababa' – by 10 months)
- disordered developmental sequence (e.g. hyperlexia coexisting with delayed language – that is, precocious reading skills well in advance of understanding)
- motor asymmetry
- qualitative concerns about emerging skills and abilities
- developmental regression – that is, loss or plateauing of skills (this is a dementia if the cause is biological, or regression if the cause is psychological).

Developmental history-taking

Parents are usually best at remembering whether or not they have had past concerns and, if so, what those concerns were. However, parents' interpretation of what their child does may reflect a wish or desire on their part rather than reality (e.g. 'he understands everything I say').

The mental health worker should taking the history should:

- use open-ended questions, followed by requests for examples, as these elicit the best history
- follow up with a specific list of closed questions to fill gaps in history
- encourage accounts of observations of behaviour rather than interpretations of motives (e.g. 'he will fetch his shoes only if they are visible')
- ask for the parental view of causation
- reassure parents as to what has not caused the child's difficulties, such as a belief that autism could be caused by the mother going out to work, or being depressed, or having agreed to immunisation with the single vaccine for measles, mumps and rubella (MMR)
- reassure parents, where appropriate, that their efforts to date have been extremely relevant, useful and productive.

Observation and interactive assessment

A suitable selection of toys should be available, covering a range of skills, interests and developmental stages and domains, such as:

- copying behaviour (bell) and understanding of cause and effect (pop-up animal toy)
- evidence of pre-verbal understanding – defining a real object by using it (cup/spoon, doll/brush) and showing symbolic understanding of the intended real-life role of play materials (doll/teddy/tea set)
- fine motor and eye–hand skills – explored with the use of coloured bricks, crayons, pencil, paper, soft ball, form boards, puzzles
- language and play (books with single pictures and stories, range of everyday toy objects, large-world and miniature-world toys).

It is helpful to have to hand toys that will appeal more to individuals at early sensory developmental stages (e.g. soft, squidgy, noisy, lighting-up) and those with obsessional/autistic tendencies (e.g. construction toys, ones with repetitive potential such as ball helter-skelters).

Most children function better when a helpful adult interacts with them, but time should be allowed for 'free play'. This is partly because children's ability to explore and organise the environment and generate ideas on their own is significant. The attending adult should not be too helpful, therefore.

The child may not be able to focus attention, flitting from one object to another. Alternatively, very repetitive play may be noted.

The mental health worker should observe not only at what child does, but also how the child does it. Thus quality of response needs monitoring as well as actual achievement.

Developmental domains

There are five developmental domains:

- gross motor
- visual behaviour (eye–hand coordination, problem-solving)
- language and communication
- play and social behaviour
- attentional behaviour.

Language and communication as contributors to emotional and behavioural disturbance

Children may be frustrated at their inability to communicate, understand and be understood. Behaviours may in themselves be forms of communication (e.g. throwing objects when child wishes to end an activity). Thus there is a high risk of the child's communication strategies being mistaken for challenging behaviours, to be snuffed out.

The parents' level of understanding of their child's communication needs is important:

- they may not understand their child's communicative behaviours
- they may communicate with the child at a level not commensurate with that child's understanding.

Children with good understanding of daily family routines, and well-developed speech, often have their language comprehension overestimated by parents.

Play and social behaviour as contributors to emotional and behavioural disturbance

The mental health worker should:

- consider the child's social development and explicitly exclude developmental disorders such as autism and hyperkinetic disorder, which may not have been considered in past assessments
- note that play, social development and attentional skills progress through developmental sequences, just as motor and language development do, and consider the child's stage of development in relation to the overall level of learning disability
- look at pro-social behaviour, including sharing, joint attention skills, including quality of eye contact used with communicative intent, pointing and other gestures.

Attention behaviour

The development of attention, concentration span and freedom from impulsiveness and distractibility, as for other skills, passes through a succession of developmental stages as skills become increasingly sophisticated and mature. There are six stages in the development of attention:

1   extreme distractibility, with attention held momentarily by whatever is the dominant stimulus (year 1)
2   concentration on task of own choice, ignoring all other things in order to focus; extreme resistance to interference by adult (year 2)
3   adult can shift child from one task to another; attention must still be fully gained before changing focus (year 3, 'single-channel attention')
4   ability to control own focus of attention; gradual move towards only needing to look at adult when directions become difficult to understand (year 4, early 'integrated attention')
5   at school entry age, ability to perform activity while listening to teacher's instructions (year 5, short periods of integrated attention)
6   mature stage, with attention flexible and sustainable for long periods.

Physical health and examination

The mental health worker should consider need for paediatric opinion if:

- there is the remotest possibility of physical symptoms
- self-injury or aggression is inexplicable
- there is plateauing or loss of physical, psychological or other developmental skills
- new onset of significant behavioural deterioration is not fully explained by the current diagnosis and assessment
- there are unusual skin signs
  - there are pigmented, hypo-pigmented or rough skin patches
  - there are capillary or cavernous haemangiomas ('naevi').

Compromised communication skills and low pain sensitivity may mask physical illness or lead to its expression through emotional and behavioural change.

Some conditions show physical signs in older childhood not present at birth or in infancy. These include:

- some forms of mucopolysaccharidoses
- adenoma sebaceum in tuberous sclerosis
- dysmorphic features – these may become more evident only in later childhood or even post-pubertally (e.g. testicular enlargement in fragile-X syndrome), or subtle signs may be missed in infancy (e.g. foetal alcohol syndrome).

Developmental diagnosis and management

The outcome of the developmental assessment will give a profile of developmental abilities and disabilities ('strengths and needs'), alongside emotional, behavioural and mental health assessments. The combined picture may indicate one or more of:

- global learning disability
- characteristic clusters of specific developmental delays or qualitative impairments (e.g. autistic-spectrum disorder, ADHD)
- specific learning difficulties (e.g. dyslexia, dyspraxia, dysarthria, dysphasia, dyscalculia, dysgraphia, sensory integration difficulties).

Laboratory investigations may be indicated to explore possible medical causes of behavioural presentations, as well as developmental disabilities and physical issues, such as:

- behavioural phenotypes (Down, fragile-X, Prader–Willi, Angelman, Lesch–Nyhan, Smith–Magenis syndromes, tuberous sclerosis, sex chromosome aneuploides and so on)
- self-injury
- aggression
- hyperkinesis and attentional deficits
- sleep disorder
- social and communicatory impairments
- epilepsy.

Further useful specialist evaluations after initial assessment include:

- speech and language therapy
- occupational therapy
- community paediatrician
- specific multidisciplinary assessment for autistic-spectrum disorder, ADHD, or psychiatric disturbances (e.g. depression, anxiety states, attachment disorder, obsessive–compulsive disorder).

Links between CAMHS and the child development services

Co-location and other strong links between teams, where possible, allows joint working, seamless services and discussion about referrals and case management.

Good care management, working together with clear and agreed multidisciplinary and multi-agency plans, named key workers and close collaboration with family and other statutory, private and voluntary agencies are necessary for the effective management of complex difficulties such as emotional and behavioural difficulties in children and young people with learning disability.

Important conditions

Foetal alcohol syndrome (alcohol-related neurodevelopmental disorder)

- Alcohol is the toxin to which a foetus is most commonly exposed.
- The syndrome features pre- and postnatal growth deficiency.
- IQ is usually in the mild/borderline learning disability range.
- There are fine-motor and visuospatial problems, including tremulousness.
- There are problems with executive function, numeracy and abstraction.
- There are expressive and receptive language difficulties.
- Irritability is seen in infancy, hyperactivity in childhood.
- There are problems perceiving social cues.
- Family environments are often very unstable, with high rates of insecure and chaotic/disorganised attachments.

Cerebral palsy

- Psychiatric disorder is present in 40% of children with cerebral palsy.
- There is no gender predominance.
- Of those with hemiplegia:
  - 25% have conduct/emotional disorder
  - 10% have hyperkinetic disorder
  - 3% have an autistic disorder.
- The best predictor of behavioural problems among those with cerebral palsy is low IQ.
- Disorders manifest identically to those of psychosocial origin.

Down syndrome

- This is the most common identifiable genetic cause of learning disability.
- Mean IQ is in moderate–severe learning disability range.
- Those with Down syndrome have a characteristic personality and temperament.
- There are relatively low rates of autistic-spectrum disorders and attention-deficit disorders in childhood.
- There are comparatively high rates of depression.
- There are comparatively high rates of Alzheimer's disease in adulthood.
- A major risk factor for Down syndrome is maternal older age.

Fragile-X syndrome

- This is the commonest identifiable inherited cause of learning disability.
- Mean IQ is in mild–moderate learning disability range.
- There are high rates of autistic-spectrum disorder and ADHD (inattentive type as well as overactive–impulsive and combined types).
- There are particular cognitive problems with sequential information processing, numeracy and visuospatial abilities.
- People with the syndrome are, characteristically, friendly and sociable, albeit shy and socially anxious, often with a range of autistic-like communicatory and ritualistic features, including delayed echolalia, rapid and dysrhythmic and repetitive speech, hand-flapping and gaze aversion.
- Male and female pre-mutation carriers show varying rates of the above difficulties.
- Female carriers experience premature ovarian failure.
- Male and female pre-mutation carriers experience middle-aged onset of tremor–ataxia syndrome with associated loss of cognitive skills.

Positive prognostic features for children and young people with learning disability who have mental health problems

Prognostic features include:

- level of intellectual functioning (the higher the better)
- presence of social awareness
- presence of meaningful language (expressive and receptive)
- presence of attentional skills
- warm, nurturing and structured family environment
- developmentally appropriate, focused and structured schooling
- progress to date.

Further reading

Cornish, K., Turk, J. & Levitas, A. (2007) Fragile X syndrome and autism: common developmental pathways? *Current Pediatric Reviews*, **3**, 61–68.

Mukherjee, R. A. S., Hollins, S. & Turk, J. (2006) Fetal alcohol spectrum disorder: an overview. *Journal of the Royal Society of Medicine*, **99**, 298–302.

Sharma, A., O'Sullivan, T. & Baird, G. (2005) Paediatric developmental assessment. *Psychiatry*, **4**, 13–18.

Turk, J. (1996) Working with parents of children who have severe learning disabilities. *Clinical Child Psychology & Psychiatry*, **1**, 581–596.

Turk, J. (2003) The importance of diagnosis (pp. 15–19), Behaviours and management (pp. 132–143), Medication matters (pp. 149–155), Support for individuals with fragile X syndrome and their families (pp. 181–187). In *Educating Children with Fragile X Syndrome* (ed. D. Dew-Hughes). Routledge Falmer.

Turk, J. (2004) Children with developmental disabilities and their parents. In *Cognitive Behaviour Therapy for Children and Families* (2nd edn) (ed. P. Graham), pp. 244–262. Cambridge University Press.

Turk, J. (2005) The mental health needs of children with learning disabilities. In *Mental Health Learning Disabilities, A Training Resource* (eds G. Holt, S. Hardy & N. Bouras). Pavilion.

Turk, J. (2007) Chromosomal abnormalities. In *Cambridge Handbook of Psychology, Health and Medicine* (2nd edn) (eds S. Ayers, A. Baum, C. McManus, *et al*), pp. 625–629. Cambridge University Press.

Turk, J. (2007) (ed. for special issue) *Advances in Mental Health in Learning Disabilities*, **1**, 1–65.

Turk, J., Graham, P. J. & Verhulst, F. (2007) *Child and Adolescent Psychiatry: A Developmental Approach* (4th edn). Oxford University Press.

CHAPTER 3

Clinical psychology

Assessment – diagnosis and degree of disability

- Clinical psychologists collaborate with other child and adolescent mental health professionals. They consider:
  - whether the child has an autistic-spectrum disorder in addition to learning disability
  - the degree and profile of learning disability
  - whether the child has ADHD.
- Differential diagnoses include specific learning difficulties, attachment disorders, language impairment and dyspraxia.
- Assessment of autistic-spectrum disorder requires home and school observation. This information is considered in conjunction with speech and language therapy and other assessments, including a thorough developmental history.
- Diagnostic decisions are aided by formal interviews (e.g. the Autism Diagnostic Interview; Lord *et al*, 2000), observation schedules (e.g. ADOS; Lord *et al*, 1994) and checklists (e.g. the Children's Communication Checklist; Bishop, 2003).
- Assessment of ADHD requires observation in various settings. Establishing the child's developmental level is important in order to consider whether problems are out of keeping with that developmental level.
- Establishing the child's level and profile of cognitive functioning can help in:
  - planning appropriate education settings
  - parents and others pitching expectations correctly
  - understanding of the child's behaviour.
- Formal cognitive assessments are complicated by attentional difficulties and many children falling below the basal level of tests. Useful assessments include:
  - Leiter–R (Roid & Miller, 1998), which can be carried out with no or limited verbal instruction

- Snijders–Ooman–R (Tellegen *et al*, 2007), which is a short (four-item) measure of non-verbal IQ requiring no spoken language on the part of either the child or the administrator.
- If direct assessment is impracticable, Vineland Adaptive Behaviour Scales (Sparrow *et al*, 1984), completed with parents/carers, provide useful information about developmental level in several domains.

Factors to consider in relation to behaviours that challenge

The most common emotional/behavioural problems presenting in children with developmental disabilities are:

- those that are developmentally related – for example, toileting (training, smearing, phobias), feeding (under-eating, over-eating or faddy eating habits), sleep (getting to sleep, night waking)
- those that challenge either because of harm to self or others or because they limit access to community facilities – for example, tantrums and aggression (towards adults, peers or property), self-harm (eye-poking, skin-picking, hair-pulling, face-slapping, head-banging) and sexualised behaviour (masturbation, inappropriate touching of others)
- those that relate to the child's emotional well-being and quality of life (withdrawn, socially isolated).

Approaches are similar to those that might be adopted with children who have no learning disability. The psychologist should:

- consider the onset of the problem and recent changes or events in the child's life, immediate triggers for the behaviour, and reinforcers for the behaviour (using ABC charts that log details of behaviour with antecedents and consequences), together with observations
- break down tasks into small steps (e.g. learning to use the toilet and learning to go to sleep alone), together with an agreed routine and reinforcers that are meaningful to the child and feasible for the family
- gather and apply existing knowledge with additions and adaptations as necessary
- take into account in the assessment three essential elements – the person, the environment, the behaviour – and interactions between these.

Factors intrinsic to the child

The psychologist should interview or play with the child and gather his or her views if possible. If this is not possible because of language and cognitive limitations, it remains important to have a sense of the child as an individual.

The psychological assessment should consider whether the child has difficulties with sensory processing. (Many children with learning disability, autistic-spectrum disorders or ADHD are hypo- or hyper-sensitive to touch, hearing, vision, smell, taste and vestibular experiences. This makes them sensation-seeking, to maintain alertness. However, they can then overload and become either difficult to calm or sensation avoidant. They may react strongly to stimuli they experience as aversive or unduly fascinating and attractive – e.g. loud noises, clothing textures, bright lights, being patted on the shoulder, strong odours, certain tastes.) Problems with sensory processing may cause behavioural difficulties. Use of the Dunn Sensory Profile (Dunn, 1999) is helpful in clarifying possible sensory issues. Interventions should be jointly planned to address challenging behaviours through therapeutic programmes to develop sensory processing abilities, or through programmes that help meet the need for sensory input in ways that do not challenge others.

There are four other points that should be considered within the psychological assessment:

- whether the child has a condition with a recognised behavioural phenotype, such as Prader–Willi syndrome (see above for further details of behavioural phenotypes)
- the child's likes and dislikes, to identify potential reinforcers and aversive stimuli
- whether the child has a psychiatric disorder such as schizophrenia, depression, cyclical mood disorder, anxiety state or obsessive–compulsive disorder
- whether the child is responding to physical discomfort, for example resulting from constipation, toothache, mouth ulcers, gastro-oesophageal reflux ('heartburn'') or otitis media (earache).

Factor intrinsic to the environment

There are three aspects of the environment to consider:

- physical environment (lighting, size, temperature, etc.)
- interpersonal environment (relationships, beliefs and values)
- organisational setting (systems in place to support the person).

The physical environment should be assessed from two points of view:

- stimulation point of view (over- or under-stimulation)
- boundary-setting and risk.

In relation to the latter, it may be more appropriate to have safety glass and door locks fitted than to increase parental stress with a behaviour programme. Is there a safe space for time-out or calm-down time? Where are keys, knives and matches kept? Can the television set, oven and other vulnerable appliances be made safe with Perspex covers, or by attaching them to the wall?

The psychological assessment should consider whether the child is engaged in activities that are over- or under-demanding. Establishing the developmental level will facilitate this. It is important to look at the rhythm of the child's day and whether the child experiences the right mix of activities (physical, stimulating, relaxing and social).

Operant learning models provide a helpful framework for behaviours that challenge. Is the child trying to escape undesirable tasks ('demand avoidance')? Is the child finding a way to obtain attention (either positive or negative)? Is the child trying to escape an unpleasant stimulus ('negative reinforcement')?

The psychologist should consider a skills-deficit approach:

- Does the carer have unrealistic expectations of the child's abilities, leading to mutual frustration?
- Does the child lack self-occupancy skills or communication channels?
- Does the child know the rules (e.g. where not to masturbate)?
- Does the child find it easier to process visual than auditory information?
- Does the child lack problem-solving skills?

Other points that should be included in the psychological assessment are:

- attachment issues
- abuse – children with learning disability are at significantly higher risk than other children of all forms of abuse, neglect and disadvantage (for refugee children it may be difficult to establish a clear history even though abuse/trauma is strongly suspected)
- the social environment –
  - do they have any friends?
  - are they able to have contact with them outside of school?
  - what is their level of self-esteem?
  - do they feel they can exert some control or make choices?
  - do they feel very different to their peers/siblings?
- the family environment and parental mental health – many parents are under substantial stress and suffer with anxiety or depression, or may have more significant mental health problems; and many families fragment and separate following the birth of a child with a disability, leaving single parents even more vulnerable to mental health problems and social disadvantage
- whether the school or play/respite setting is appropriate to the child's needs.

It may be that the behaviour is the only way for the child to communicate. What supports are in place to aid more appropriate communication? If it is possible to teach more appropriate ways of communicating (e.g. using Makaton or a 'picture exchange communication symbol', or PECS), then the behaviour (e.g. a tantrum) may diminish. Visual timetables, communication passports and social stories are all useful techniques.

Factors intrinsic to the behaviour

Behaviours should be described in detail. The psychologist should:

- investigate the onset, severity, duration and frequency of the behaviour
- establish a baseline measure of the behaviour, so that the effectiveness of any intervention can be measured
- establish how others responded when the behaviour first appeared.

Direct observation is important, as are the observations of those in contact with the child.

Interventions

Direct work

- It can be effective to work with the child to build skills in identifying and naming different feeling states with the use of words, symbols, gestures, or pictorial representations of different feeling states, even if the child is non-verbal. Interventions should be concrete and use strategies that appeal to the child's interests (e.g. an 'anger volcano' made out of clay, bicarbonate of soda and vinegar to track the feelings as they build; or a traffic light system or penalty card system).
- Communication issues will arise. It may not be possible for the mental health worker to become sufficiently accomplished in Makaton or other alternative and augmentative communication methods. However, there will usually be someone who knows the child well who is an expert on how the child is communicating and they should be asked for guidance; it may even be desirable for the CAMHS to work through that person.
- Direct work can be either home based or school based. This will need to be decided.
- Life-story work can be useful where there has been loss or change. This may take the form of an 'All About Me' book, with photographs of people, places and activities that form the basis for discussion and exploration of personal feelings.
- Cognitive–behavioural methods are of proven efficacy. Children's cognitive abilities and whether they can differentiate emotions need to be considered.
- Adolescence poses new issues for the individual and family. Systemic family work can be of value.
- Transitions are particularly stressful times (e.g. starting nursery, a new school, moving home).

Risk assessment and reactive strategies

- In instances of challenging behaviour, risk should be assessed.
- Reactive strategies aim to ensure the safety of the person who is challenging and those in his or her vicinity. They are not designed to produce long-term behavioural changes. They should be used in conjunction with a broader behaviour programme and preventive strategies.
- Reactive strategies should follow the principle of least intrusiveness and least restrictiveness (e.g. ignoring behaviour, leaving the scene, distracting the child).
- Any indicators that the risky behaviour is about to occur and any patterns of escalation in behaviour need to be noted.
- Any reactive strategies that may reinforce the challenging behaviour in the longer term should be avoided.
- Where physical interventions may be necessary, these should be used as infrequently as possible. When they are used, this should be only in the best interests of the child. Restrictive physical interventions should be seen as one part of a broader strategy to address the needs of children whose behaviour poses a serious challenge to services and carers. Specialist training is essential if holding techniques are to be employed.

Problems occurring at network level

Children with disabilities quickly become the joint 'concern' of various people in the systems that surround them. This provides numerous opportunities for disagreement, splitting, breakdowns in communication and falling through the net. The system is complex, covering primary, secondary and tertiary levels of care in both acute and community sectors of the health service, various sections of the education department, social services, and community and voluntary agencies. Even professionals can find it hard to keep up to date with services available and current procedures, and parents need support in negotiating this system.

Professionals may play a role when the child's school placement is under threat or has permanently broken down. Can the challenging behaviour be modified? Can the professional provide a neutral space for the parent to consider future options, including the possibility of the child going to residential school? Can the professional provide information to others in the network or to the parents that makes expectations more realistic?

Psychologists working at network level should take into account the following points:

- Work should be holistic.
- Are parental mental health issues affecting effective functioning of

the support system around the child? Can joint work with the adult mental health service promote improvements here?

- Many siblings of children with disabilities are profoundly affected. Can they be referred on for support, both practical (e.g. homework clubs, young carers' play schemes) and therapeutic (individual and family work)?
- The impact of any lack of appropriate play, transport, medical and respite services needs to be considered. This is likely to be especially relevant where the family's finances are stretched (many parents are unable to work because of their child's needs).
- The effect of care provided by unskilled foster carers may need to be considered, in which case the psychologist may be able to work together with them creatively, flexibly and jointly to offer a local solution.
- Many families present at transition points in the child's life. Families need additional support from the network to negotiate these times.
- The psychologist's approach needs to be flexible and at times overlap with what traditionally might be the role of another professional.

How might the psychologist's role differ from that when working with children who do not have a learning disability?

- Psychologists may do very little clinic-based work to ensure engagement and efficacy.
- There is a lot more liaison, which is essential but time-consuming.
- Negotiating confidentiality issues can be different and complex since psychologists may work in a team dedicated to children with disabilities where it is common practice to share information about both individuals and organisations.
- It is very practical.
- Psychologists need to be flexible when thinking about what their role might be.
- They may do work over the telephone, via email, in schools, homes and elsewhere to ensure accessibility and engagement.
- The work tends to be long term but it is not endless and families can come to feel empowered and skilled enough to manage with infrequent input.
- Systemic ideas (Baum & Lynggaard, 2006) are useful but not used in a purist manner. They are used to consider the system and the child's, family's and problem's position within it.
- Cognitive–behavioural therapy is useful but will need to be adapted and used alongside other concrete and non-verbal techniques in one-to-one work.

- Psychologists may be limited in what they can provide because of policies, procedures or politics in the system surrounding the child and they may need to think in supervision how senior managers can take these issues up and develop a more facilitative milieu for interventions to succeed. For example, with children over 16, can senior managers negotiate the use of adult learning disability services? Can a working party be set up between the social work team, the local education authority and CAMHS to consider the needs of children excluded from school?

Further reading

Baum, S. & Lynggaard, H. (2006) *Intellectual Disabilities – A Systemic Approach.* Karnac.

Bishop, D. (2003) *Children's Communication Checklist – Second Edition (CCC2).* Pearson Education.

Clements, J. & Martin, N. (2002) *Assessing Behaviours Regarded as Problematic in People with Developmental Disabilities.* Jessica Kingsley.

Dunn, W. (1999) *Sensory Profile.* Pearson.

Emerson, E. (2001) *Challenging Behaviour: Analysis and Intervention in People with Severe Intellectual Disabilities* (2nd edn). Cambridge University Press.

Lord, C., Rutter, M. & Le Couteur, A. (1994) Autism Diagnostic Interview – Revised: a revised version of a diagnostic interview for caregivers of individuals with possible pervasive developmental disorders. *Journal of Autism & Developmental Disorders,* **24,** 659–685.

Lord, C., Risi, S., Lambrecht, L., *et al* (2000) The Autism Diagnostic Observation Schedule—Generic: a standard measure of social and communication deficits associated with the spectrum of autism. *Journal of Autism & Developmental Disorders,* **30,** 205–223.

Roid, G. & Miller, L. (1998) *Leiter International Performance Scale – Revised.* GL Assessment.

Sparrow, S., Balla, D. & Cicchetti, D. (1984) *The Vineland Adaptive Behavior Scales.* nferNelson.

Tellegen, P. J. Winkel, M. & Laros J. A. (2007) *SON-R – Snijders-Oomen Non-Verbal Intelligence Test (Revised) 2.5–7 Years* (3rd version, UK adaptation). Hogrefe UK.

Turk, J. (2004) Children with developmental disabilities and their parents. In *Cognitive Behaviour Therapy for Children and Families* (2nd edn) (ed. P. Graham), pp. 244–262. Cambridge University Press.

Turk, J. & O'Brien, G. (2002) Counselling parents and carers of individuals with behavioural phenotypes. In *Behavioural Phenotypes in Clinical Practice* (ed. G. O'Brien), pp. 152–168. MacKeith Press.

CHAPTER 4

Speech and language therapy

Approaches to the assessment of language and communication within speech and language therapy (SLT) tend to be similar for all individuals. Intervention is based on findings from assessment which differ for each client. Some SLT contributions are specific to in-patient or out-patient settings, while others are applicable to both. An ideal speech and language therapy programme should:

- be tailored to individual needs
- have aims incorporated into all daily activities and all social situations
- be available 24 hours a day, 7 days a week, 365 days a year
- be developed, monitored and modified by speech and language therapists
- be carried out by those with most regular contact with the child, *having been trained to do so by a speech and language therapist.*

Epidemiology

- Twenty-three per cent of 5- to 8-year-olds referred to psychiatry out-patient departments have unsuspected moderate or severe language disorder (Cohen *et al*, 1998)
- Of 17 children aged 6–12 years in a unit for children with emotional and behavioural difficulties, 16 presented with speech or language problems (or both) requiring SLT intervention (Burgess & Bransby, 1990)
- In one study, 60% of pre-adolescents in psychiatric hospital had significant speech and language problems, but only 38% had ever received SLT (Giddan & Ross, 1997).

Nature of speech and language impairment in individuals who have learning disability

Speech and language impairment in individuals who have learning disability may be:

- part of the general picture of developmental delay
- characteristic of a particular condition or syndrome
- a distinct additional impairment.

Assessment

- The therapist contacts community teams and SLT colleagues to collect data on communication status, previous assessments and interventions, and collates and summarises these.
- SLT assessment takes a holistic view of the individual, placing language and communication skills in a broad context. Interactions with behaviour, social skills and educational attainment are critical.
- Areas of investigation should include:
  - pragmatic skills (context, use, appropriateness, relevance, conversation, discourse)
  - semantics (meaning, vocabulary)
  - syntax (grammar, sentences)
  - speech (phonology, articulation and phonological awareness)
  - literacy (reading and spelling).
- Investigation in each area should include assessment of verbal and non-verbal:
  - input (hearing, seeing, attention, listening, looking)
  - processing (understanding, sorting, ordering, thinking, remembering)
  - output (speech, vocabulary, sentences, narrative, fluency, behaviour).
- Sources of information should include the effect of language and communication skills on emotional and behavioural functioning, and should be considered from multiple perspectives and in multiple environmental contexts.
- Standardised assessments help professionals to compare language skills against those of the 'normal' population and highlight areas of strength and weakness. The limitations of such instruments with this client group must be acknowledged, however.
- Observations by speech and language therapists, CAMHS staff and carers in different settings provide essential information on a person's ability to utilise language and communication skills in different contexts (e.g. structured, educational, social).
- Questionnaires and profiles provide a structured format for gathering information and considering certain patterns of behaviour.
- The impact of level of language and communication skills should be considered in relation to:
  - functional communication (effect of language disability on daily life, including self/other awareness, organisation, interaction, learning, autonomy, choice)

- relationships
- behaviour (antecedents, communicative intent, consequences)
- higher-level language functioning (verbal reasoning, problem-solving, making predictions, inferences, etc.).

Intervention

- Speech and language therapists use a range of service delivery methods to suit clients' needs and chosen intervention. These include:
  - consultation, with the multidisciplinary team, carers and other professionals
  - direct intervention with the individual in group or one-to-one settings
  - indirect intervention through another person, such as a member of the support staff or a carer
  - collaboration to identify needs, solve problems and develop interventions
  - client-centred training packages (e.g. training carers)
  - environmental change (e.g. use of visual cues, changes in language levels used).
- The intervention should:
  - acknowledge individual strengths and needs to address areas of weakness, starting at the difficulty's source (i.e. input, processing or output)
  - take into account available time and resources.
- The therapist should:
  - advise carers and other professionals as to the appropriate language level to be used with the individual and any environmental changes required (e.g. picture cues, colour coding)
  - alert carers and other professionals to potential difficulties relating to interactions between language and behaviour
  - choose from a range of available theoretical approaches and interventions
  - closely monitor the efficacy of the intervention.
- The intervention frequently begins with development of awareness of self or others to orientate the individual to the reciprocal nature of communication, as is done with the 'I Am Special' (Vermeulen, 2000) and 'Talkabout' approaches (Kelly, 2001).
- The development of functional literacy skills is important, as it allows the child to access education and to develop vocabulary and higher-level language skills. Therapists have a role in developing phonological and language skills required for acquisition of literacy.
- Individuals benefit from learning strategies that address their own communication breakdown, and that recognise their vulnerable areas

in both understanding and language use (Dollaghan and Kaston, 1986).

- Direct teaching of thinking skills can facilitate learning and organisation of other knowledge, as is done with 'Mind Maps' (Hoffman, 2001; Buzan & Buzan, 2006) and 'Thinking Hats' (de Bono, 2000).

- Individuals with poor understanding or expressive use of vocabulary will benefit from multi-modal and multi-sensory approaches to learning new words with large numbers of repetitions, for example using semantic links (Lewis & Speake, 1993).

- Narrative is an effective method of improving functional language and discourse skills in children and adolescents (Joffe, 2006; Stringer, 2006).

- When teaching social skills, it is essential that individuals have appropriate language modelled for them and opportunities to practise using language in a variety of contexts.

- Alternative and augmentative communication methods may be required, either as a temporary support to the development of spoken language or as a permanent means of communication. These can be high- or low-technology. Examples include:
  - signing (e.g. Makaton)
  - symbol use (e.g. Boardmaker, Blissymbolics)
  - visual timetables, schedules (e.g. TEACCH)
  - talking mats
  - voice output aids.

References

Burgess, J. & Bransby, G. (1990) An evaluation of the speech and language skills of children with emotional and behavioural problems. *CSLT Bulletin*, January, 2–3.

Buzan, T. & Buzan, B. (2006) *The Mind Map Book*. Ashford Colour Press.

Cohen, N. J., Barwick, M., Horodezky, N. B., *et al* (1998) Language achievement and cognitive processing in psychiatrically disturbed children with previously identified and unsuspected language impairments. *Journal of Child Psychology and Psychiatry*, **39**, 865–877.

De Bono, E. (2000) *Six Thinking Hats* (2nd revised edn). Penguin Books.

Dollaghan, C. & Kaston, N. (1986) A comprehension monitoring program for language-impaired children. *Journal of Speech and Hearing Disorders*, **51**, 264–271.

Giddan, J. & Ross, G. (1997) Selective mutism in elementary school: multidisciplinary interventions. *Language, Speech and Hearing Services in Schools*, **28**, 127–133.

Hoffman, E. (2001) *Introducing Children to Mind Mapping*. Learn to Learn.

Joffe, V. (2006). Enhancing language and communication in secondary school-aged children. In *Language and Social Disadvantage* (eds J. Ginsborg & J. Clegg), pp. 207–216. John Wiley.

Kelly, A. (2001) *TALKABOUT*. Speechmark Publishing.

Lewis, S. & Speake, J. (1993) *Semantic Links*. Stass Publications.

Stringer, H. (2006) Facilitating narrative and social skills in secondary school students with language and behaviour difficulties. In *Language and Social Disadvantage* (eds J. Ginsborg & J. Clegg), pp. 199–206. John Wiley.

Taylor, C. (2004) Speech and language therapy. In *Educating Children with Fragile X Syndrome: A Multiprofessional View* (ed. D. Dew-Hughes), pp. 106–114. Routledge Falmer.

Vermeulen, P. (2000) *I Am Special*. Jessica Kingsley.

CHAPTER 5

Occupational therapy

The aim of occupational therapy is to help children become as independent as possible in everyday activities and to reach their maximum functional potential. Occupational therapy considers the impact of physical, emotional and social disabilities and impairments across a range of performance areas, particularly:

- self-care (e.g. dressing and personal hygiene)
- learning (e.g. school-based tasks)
- play and leisure (e.g. taking part in community activities).

Occupational therapists

Occupational therapists are concerned with enabling children and young people to master skills necessary for daily life (as above). These skills involve an interplay between personal characteristics, cultural setting and motor, sensory, cognitive and social abilities.

Paediatric occupational therapists work with children (from newborn through adolescence) whose rate of growth, development and maturation is interrupted as a result of any physical, social, emotional or learning disability, trauma, deprivation or disease.

Occupational therapists work with children and their families, focusing on the person–environment–occupation interface (Table 5.1), within all models of practice, in order to support children's ability to fulfil their everyday occupations and roles.

Occupational therapy assessment

Different frames of reference, incorporating a range of assessment tools, may be used to determine how and why problems occur in performance and adaptive behaviour and to identify mechanisms for intervention (McElderry, 2000).

Table 5.1 Areas of assessment and intervention in occupational therapy

Person	Environmental	Occupational performance
Balance, posture/sitting balance, head control	Architecture/design	Daily living skills (e.g. dressing, self-care, eating)
Range of motion, movement coordination	Lighting, surfaces, access	Play/leisure
Fine manipulative skills	Attitudes	School/academic tasks (e.g. writing, using science equipment)
Sensation: touch, motion, taste, smell	Educational policies/ provision	Mobility
Endurance/strength/pacing	Housing	Money management
Mood/motivation	Transportation	Community skills
Fitness	Adaptations for weather	
Cognition (attention, planning, error detection, etc.)		
Learning and memory		
Pain, continence		

Sensory processing, including responsiveness to sensory stimulation

- There is evidence that individuals with learning disabilities, attention-deficit disorders and pervasive developmental disorders have atypical sensory processing, which may contribute to self-stimulatory or self-injurious actions in some (Tomchek & Dunn, 2007).
- Sensory modulation disorders are impairments in regulating the degree, intensity and nature of responses to sensory input, resulting in substantial problems with daily roles and routines. Some 40–80% of people with developmental disabilities have sensory modulation disorders (Baranek et al, 2002).
- Children with tactile sensitivity and poor tactile discrimination show poorer fine manipulative skills.

Sensorimotor coordination and hand function

Children with learning disabilities may have problems with balance, posture/sitting and movement control, to the detriment of their gross and fine motor abilities.

Perceptual processing

Visual spatial and visual motor abilities are associated with fine motor skills and independence in daily activities.

Problem-solving

Children with learning difficulties often have difficulties generating strategies for learning new skills and automating motor actions in the learning of a new sequence.

Psychosocial skills

- Problems with self-regulation have been associated with sensory modulation disorders.
- Children with anxiety have been shown to be at greater risk of balance and movement difficulties, and vice versa.
- There is a high incidence of coordination difficulties in children with learning and social impairments.

Occupational therapy intervention

Independence in daily activities

Community occupational therapy – through social services provision, consisting of the provision of equipment, minor and major adaptations and advice – has been shown to be effective in improving independence in children and young people.

Fine motor and functional performance

Occupational therapy for preschool children that emphasises play-based activities has been shown to improve both fine motor skills and peer interaction. Visual motor and functional outcomes are influenced by the number of sessions and percentage of sessions that specifically address self-care goals.

Sensory processing and adaptive behaviour

Occupational therapy using a sensory integration approach may be effective in improving self-regulation and adaptive behaviour and reducing self-stimulatory and self-injurious behaviour, for some young people with sensory modulation disorders.

Cognitive strategy generation for motor and social tasks

Children with mild learning disabilities or pervasive developmental disorders benefit from intervention using the 'cognitive orientation to daily occupational performance' (CO–OP) approach (Ward & Rodger, 2004) in terms of their ability and confidence in tasks involving motor skills.

References

Baranek, G. T., Chin, Y. H., Hess, L. J., *et al* (2002) Sensory processing correlates of occupational performance in children with Fragile X syndrome. *American Journal of Occupational Therapy*, **56**, 538–546.

McElderry, F. (2000) A guide to occupational therapy with children. *Current Paediatrics*, **10**, 67–71.

Tomchek, S. D. & Dunn, W. (2007) Sensory processing in children with and without autism: a comparative study using the Short Sensory Profile. *American Journal of Occupational Therapy*, **61**, 190–200.

Ward, A. & Rodger, S. (2004) The applicaiton of cognitive orientation to daily occupational performance (CO–OP) with children 5–7 years with developmental coordination disorder. *British Journal of Occupational Therapy*, **67**, 256–264.

CHAPTER 6

Nursing

As with all professions working within a CAMHS, the traditional role of a nurse is not always applicable. Most nurses will have knowledge and skills above and beyond those usually deemed to be 'nursing'. This expanded brief is sometimes referred to as the 'enhanced role'. Relevant skills can be grouped as:

- those generally applicable to all child and adolescent mental health learning disability clinicians
- those more specific to the nursing role:
  - general
  - child and adolescent
  - mental health
  - learning disability
- those representing interests specific to the individual:
  - family work
  - liaison and consultation
  - functional behavioural analysis and behaviour modification.

There is overlap between what nurses provide in CAMHS and what is provided by other common CAMHS clinicians, in particular psychologists, social workers and occupational therapists.

All nurses are individual and will bring with them knowledge and skills that interest them and that are needed or are not forthcoming from other team members. However, many nurses (trained in either learning disability or mental health) do not have the opportunity to work with children, particularly children with learning disability, during their training. Thus their specialist knowledge and skills are frequently acquired after registration.

Learning disability nursing

- Nurses working in child and adolescent mental health learning disability services may be qualified in mental health, learning disability or both.

- They are the only professional group to train solely to work with people who have learning disability.
- Training in learning disability nursing has a life-span approach, which is useful in terms of understanding and assisting with transition phases in people's lives.
- Training in nursing facilitates an understanding of the physical and complex health needs of people with learning disability.
- Behavioural theory and practice are part of training for learning disability nursing.
- Learning disability nurse training and clinical practice have a bio-psychosocial approach.
- The ability to work in in-patient, out-patient and a wide range of outreach settings is integral to nursing practice within child and adolescent mental health learning disability.

Core areas of learning disability nursing practice

Nurses have a key role in each of the following areas:

- assessment of need
- health surveillance and health promotion
- developing personal competence (skill-building)
- enhanced therapeutic skills
- managing and leading teams of staff.

Learning disability nurses within a CAMHS

Within a CAMHS, nurses undertake:

- multi-modal assessments
- a bio-psychosocial approach to assessment, intervention and support
- comprehensive and detailed behavioural assessments, including functional assessment, analogue behavioural ratings, functional analysis, and construction and monitoring of behaviour modification programmes (many nurses have a good grounding in cognitive approaches as well)
- work across disciplines and across agencies
- the development, implementation and evaluation of comprehensive care plans
- the implementation of comprehensive treatment packages, particularly ones relating to challenging needs
- a hands-on approach often lacking from other disciplines
- the inclusion and involvement of clients and families in assessment and treatment.

CHAPTER 7

The social work contribution

The social work report

It is important to establish the authority to write a social work report. All qualified social workers should be registered with the General Social Care Council (GSCC). The title 'social worker" has been protected by law in England since 1 April 2005. This law came from the Care Standards Act 2000 to ensure that only those who are properly qualified, registered and accountable for their work describe themselves as social workers.

Registration ensures that those working in social care meet rigorous registration requirements and will be held to account for their conduct by codes of practice. Qualifications, health and good character are checked as part of the registration process. Registered social workers are also required to complete post-registration training and learning activities before renewing their registration every three years. Further information can be found at http://www.gscc.org.uk.

Since 2000, social work and social work reports have been guided by the 'framework for assessment' (see below) and social workers have been encouraged to develop evidenced-based practice.

Framework for assessment

The key principles guiding the social work assessment (and report) are as follows (see also Fig. 9.1):

- It is child centred.
- It is rooted in child development (which includes recognition of the significance of timing in a child's life).
- It takes an ecological approach, locating the child within the family and the wider community.
- It is based on ensuring equality of opportunity for all children and their families.

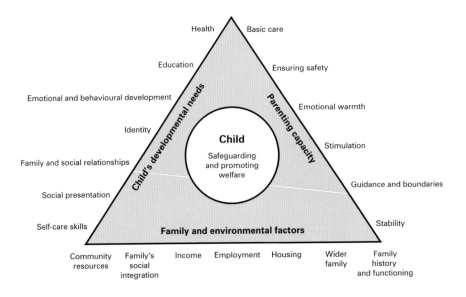

Fig. 7.1 The framework for social work assessment.

- It is based on working in partnership with families and young people.
- It builds on the strengths in each of the three domains of the child, parents and family/environmental factors.
- It is a multi-agency approach model in which it is not just social care departments that are the assessors and providers of services.
- Assessment is seen as a process, not a single event.
- Action and services should be provided in parallel with assessment, according to the needs of the child and family – not awaiting the 'completion of assessment'.
- It is grounded in knowledge derived from theory, research, policy and practice.

There are, however, other dimensions that need to be taken into consideration when preparing a social work report for a child with a learning disability.

Communication

Children may have particular needs, especially in relation to communication, which must be addressed to make any assessment meaningful. It is the responsibility of the social worker to ensure that the child has the best possible chance of communicating. This may mean: learning about each individual child's method; using interpreters or facilitators; tuning to non-verbal communication techniques; or thinking creatively about ways of listening.

Parenting

Where a child's needs are complex, assessments of parenting capacity can be particularly challenging. Some children need more parenting or more skilled parenting than others; some children need intensive parenting for much longer than others. Caring for a child with a learning disability makes emotional, physical, social, time and financial demands on parents and carers that go well beyond what is expected of parents of children who have no disability. The task of caring for a child with complex needs may be more complicated, more time-consuming, less familiar, more anxiety-provoking, physically more challenging, and emotionally more difficult.

Support networks

Social workers should explore more widely the context in which the child lives. Supports available to most parents are often less available to parents of children with learning disabilities. Those supports that are available are often scarce, cost more and often mean joining a waiting list. The risk of family breakdown is higher, and baby-sitting, respite, leisure pursuits and other informal supports may be much harder to find.

Equality issues

The cultural identity of children with a learning disability needs active recognition. The situation of black and other ethnic minority children with learning disabilities requires particular attention, because the effects of racism and disablism can compound each other. Research demonstrates that families from minority ethnic groups caring for children with a disability are even more disadvantaged that white families in similar situations.

CHAPTER 8

Medical

Children and young people with learning disability who have mental health problems often do not meet the diagnostic criteria for a specific psychiatric disorder. Instead, they present with behaviour suggestive of psychiatric disorder that often overlaps several diagnostic categories, fitting none of them exactly. Furthermore, indications for medications often differ from those in general CAMHS work. This chapter reviews the drugs used for ADHD, anxiety, obsessive–compulsive disorder, mood disorders, psychoses, aggression, self-injurious behaviour, sleep disorder and tics. Psychotropic medications are often not licensed for children and young people and are rarely licensed for those with learning and other developmental disabilities. This does not mean they cannot be prescribed; in fact, many are relatively safe and potentially highly beneficial when used with this patient group (Medicines Act 1968 and the EC Pharmaceutical Directive 89/341/EEC).

Attention-deficit hyperactivity disorder

- It is first necessary to consider whether the behaviour is compatible with the child's developmental level; inattention and overactivity are more common in children with learning disability.
- ADHD is more common in young people with learning disability than in the general population.
- Methylphenidate (Ritalin, Equasym) is the most commonly used medication.
  - Side-effects include abdominal pain, headaches, appetite and weight loss, anxiety, agitation, insomnia, psychosis, tics, mood lability, increases in pulse rate and blood pressure, lowering of seizure threshold and reversible growth failure.
  - Height, weight, pulse and blood pressure should be monitored.
  - Long-term treatment should be anticipated if the response is good. Graded-release preparations (Concerta XL, Equasym XL, Medikinet) could be considered.

- Dexamphetamine may help when methylphenidate has proved unsuccessful or when it has produced unacceptable adverse effects.
- Atomoxetine, a selective noradrenaline reuptake inhibitor, is licensed in children and adults but is more expensive than methylphenidate or dexamphetamine.
    - It is not used routinely as a first-line treatment except when there are clinically significant problems with psychostimulants such as low weight, very poor appetite or sleep, tics, seizures, substance misuse or parents being strongly against use of stimulants.
    - Side-effects include nausea, vomiting, urinary hesitancy, rashes, weight loss, low mood, suicidal thoughts or actions (though these are rare) and hepatic failure (very rare).
- Clonidine, an α-agonist, can be beneficial, does not affect appetite and if anything promotes sleep. The initial dose is 25 μg twice daily, which may, if necessary, be increased in 25 μg increments up to a maximum of 150 μg twice daily.
- Neuroleptics are prescribed occasionally for 'hyperactivity' despite being unlicensed for this indication. Low-dose risperidone (commencing with 0.25 mg once or twice daily) can be helpful *in extremis*.
- There is a small amount of clinically anecdotal literature supporting the use of tricyclic antidepressants and SSRIs for ADHD.

Anxiety

- Most individuals with anxiety do not require pharmacological intervention. Cognitive, behavioural and social interventions are the treatments of choice.
- Pharmacotherapy should be used cautiously because of side-effects.
- If drugs are necessary to control acute anxiety, then short-acting benzodiazepines such as lorazepam and midazolam are recommended. Longer-acting agents such as diazepam cause more daytime sedation and hangover.
- SSRIs are the pharmacological treatment of choice for refractory anxiety.
- Buspirone has been used successfully in people with learning disability to reduce anxiety and related behavioural disturbance (Ratey *et al*, 1991).
- Beta-blockers may be useful for individuals who show sympathetic overactivity when emotionally aroused.

Obsessive–compulsive disorder

- Clomipramine and other SSRIs are beneficial.
- Fluvoxamine and sertraline are licensed for children and adolescents with obsessive–compulsive disorder.

Mood disorders

- Early identification and multi-modal treatment may prevent unnecessary duration of a mood disorder and progression to refractory states.
- SSRIs should be used. Problems with concentration, continence or motor coordination may arise with the use of other antidepressants (e.g. tricyclics and monoamine oxidase inhibitors).
- Lithium is helpful for bipolar mood disorders but requires diligent monitoring for possible side-effects, including polyuria with incontinence, gastrointestinal disturbance, hypothyroidism and dermatitis. It should be discontinued if there is neurotoxicity, including seizures (not due to pre-existing epilepsy), severe tremor, vomiting, lethargy and coma.
- Anticonvulsants (carbamazepine, sodium valproate, lamotrigine) are useful for children and young people. They reduce blood sampling requirements, are relatively safe and can be beneficial for cyclical (and even not so cyclical) mood and behaviour disorders.
- Atypical antipsychotics can provide or contribute to mood stabilisation.
- The combination of an antipsychotic and a mood stabiliser can help in refractory cases.

Schizophrenia and other childhood psychoses

- The first-line treatment should be an 'atypical' antipsychotic agent, such as risperidone, amisulpiride, olanzapine or quetiapine.
- Their side-effects include appetite stimulation and weight gain, sedation, movement disorder and an increase prolactin level (Table 7.1).
- A history of epilepsy should always be sought. Epilepsy affects approximately a third of children and young people with moderate to

Table 7.1 Side-effects of antipsychotic agents

Weight gain	Increased levels of prolactin	Sedation	Extrapyramidal effects
Clozapine	Risperidone	Quetiapine	Haloperidol
Olanzapine	Amisulpiride	Clozapine	Amisulpiride
Risperidone	Haloperidol	Olanzapine	Risperidone
Quetiapine	Olanzapine	Risperidone	Olanzapine
Amisulpiride	Quetiapine	Amisulpiride	Quetiapine
Aripiprazole	Clozapine	Haloperidol	Clozapine
Ziprazidone			

profound learning disability and antipsychotic medications are known to lower the convulsive threshold.

- Clozapine can be used in refractory instances but requires careful blood count monitoring for possible bone marrow suppression.
- Anticholinergic drugs to counter movement disorders should be considered when high doses of antipsychotics are prescribed, or when extrapyramidal reactions or other adverse effects persist even after the dosage of antipsychotic medication has been decreased.

Aggression

- Underlying causes of aggression such as psychiatric disorder, physical pathology with associated pain and distress, epilepsy, post-traumatic stress disorder, bereavement, abuse, neglect or other unfavourable and adverse environmental factors should always be considered and addressed if present.
- The psychological impact of extreme puzzlement, anxiety and confusion associated with autistic social, communicatory and ritualistic features must always be borne in mind.
- Antipsychotics have been used to treat aggression but their cost–benefit ratio remains unclear because of frequent side-effects.
- Risperidone can improve behavioural problems, including aggression (McCracken et al, 2002; Shea et al, 2004).
- If weight gain on risperidone is a clinically significant problem try amisulpiride or aripiprazole.
- These powerful medications should usually be prescribed under the supervision of a consultant psychiatrist trained in paediatric psychopharmacology as it relates to children and young people with developmental disabilities. Careful bio-psychosocial assessment and formulation before prescribing is required to ensure appropriate screening and monitoring.
- Height, weight, pulse, blood pressure, possible sexual side-effects, behavioural changes, extrapyramidal symptoms, bowel habit alterations and bladder disturbance should be monitored regularly.
- If a child is more than 10 centile points above the expected weight, fasting blood glucose, lipids and prolactin concentrations should be measured, to help prevent illness associated with excessive weight, following discussion on risk–benefit analysis with carers.
- Propranolol, a beta-blocker, may be of benefit for aggression.
- Carbamazepine, sodium valproate, lamotrigine and topiramate have been identified as being potentially useful for aggression.
- SSRIs may be useful in preventing aggression, through the treatment of anxiety and impulsivity.
- Buspirone is reportedly useful in decreasing aggression (Ratey et al, 1991), particularly in relation to arousal and anxiety.

- Where ADHD underlies aggression, stimulant medication may be indicated.
- Quick-acting benzodiazepine drugs can be used to treat acute aggressive episodes, but caution is needed with regard to habituation, tolerance and addiction in the medium to long term.

Self-injurious behaviour

- The extreme distress of severe self-injury, for sufferer and observers alike, results in frequent requests for medication.
- Treatment targets should be sensible and candid, especially when dealing with persistent or entrenched behaviour.
- Neurochemical hypotheses centre largely on the roles of dopamine, serotonin and endogenous opioids (King, 2000).
- Risperidone can be effective and well tolerated for the treatment of self-injurious behaviour in children with autistic disorder (McCracken *et al*, 2002).
- SSRIs can be used, especially if self-injury appears to be associated with depressive, anxiety or obsessive–compulsive features.
- A trial of naltrexone, an opioid antagonist, may be of use in preventing potentially reinforcing endogenous opioid effects in response to self-injury.
- There have been reports of success with buspirone for children who deliberately injure themselves (Verhoeven & Tuinier, 1996).
- Carbamazepine has also been described as being of potential benefit (Deb *et al*, 2008).

Sleep disorder

- Sleep hygiene measures, bedtime routines, social and environmental factors, and psychological treatments (cognitive–behavioural) should be used first with those suffering with sleep disorders.
- The use of any stimulants (caffeine, food colourings and flavourings, but also excessive television or computer time) should be minimised.
- Melatonin can be beneficial, especially for difficulties with sleep induction.
  - It is administered 20–30 minutes before the desired bedtime, initially at a low dose (e.g. 1–3 mg), which may be increased in 0.5–3 mg increments.
  - Tolerance and habituation have been reported, but these respond to drug holidays.
- Clonidine may be beneficial for repeated night-time waking, including insomnia aggravated by stimulant medication.

- Early-morning waking should trigger exploration for possible depressive disorder. If the latter is present, cognitive–behavioural therapy or an SSRI is indicated.

Tics

- Child and carer education and reassurance are the most important treatments.
- Antipsychotics (risperidone, sulpiride, pimozide) are most commonly used for tic suppression (see above for side-effect profiles).
- The lowest possible dose, at bedtime, should be used (two divided doses may give better control through the day).
- Haloperidol has prominent side-effects, some potentially long term and irreversible, and is therefore contraindicated.
- Occasionally individuals benefit from clonidine, and experience minimal side-effects.
  - Treatment with clonidine begins with 0.025–0.05 mg/day, increased in increments of 0.025–0.05 mg/day every 5–7 days.
  - Adverse effects of clonidine include sedation, cognitive blunting, irritability, headaches, decreased salivation and, at higher doses, hypotension and dizziness.
- Higher doses of neuroleptics and clonidine are not necessarily more effective but are more frequently associated with sedation.
- Reducing dosage can produce benefit where higher doses have failed.

Further reading

Danielyan, A. & Kowatch, R. A. (2005) Management options for bipolar disorder in children and adolescents. *Paediatric Drugs*, **7**, 277–294.

Deb, S., Chaplin, R., Sohanpal, S., *et al* (2008) The effectiveness of mood stabilizers and antiepileptic medication for the management of behaviour problems in adults with intellectual disability: a systematic review. *Journal of Intellectual Disability Research*, **52**, 107–113.

Gillberg, C. (ed.) (2000) Child and adolescent psychopharmacology. *European Child and Adolescent Psychiatry*, **9**, supplement 1, 1–122.

Green, W. H. (2001) *Child and Adolescent Clinical Psychopharmacology*. Lippincott, Williams and Wilkins.

Ingrassia, A. & Turk, J. (2005) The use of clonidine for severe and intractable sleep problems in children with neurodevelopmental disorders: a case series. *European Child and Adolescent Psychiatry*, **14**, 34–40.

King, B. H. (2000) Pharmacological treatment of mood disturbances, aggresssion, and self-injury in persons with pervasive developmental disorders. *Journal of Autism & Developmental Disorders*, **30**, 439–445.

McCracken, J. T., McGough, J., Shah, B., *et al* (2002) Risperidone in children with autism and serious behavioral problems. *New England Journal of Medicine*, **347**, 314–321.

Morgan, S. & Taylor, E. (2007) Antipsychotic drugs in children with autism. *BMJ*, **334**, 1069–1070.

Pearson, D. A., Santos, C. W., Roache, J. D., *et al* (2003) Treatment effects of methylphenidate on behavioral adjustment in children with mental retardation and ADHD. *Journal of the American Academy of Child and Adolescent Psychiatry*, **42**, 209–216.

Pearson, D. A., Santos, C. W., Casat, C. D., *et al* (2004a) Treatment effects of methylphenidate on cognitive functioning in children with mental retardation and ADHD. *Journal of the American Academy of Child and Adolescent Psychiatry*, **43**, 677–685.

Pearson, D. A., Lane, D. M., Santos, C. W., *et al* (2004b) Effects of methylphenidate treatment in children with mental retardation and ADHD: individual variation in medication response. *Journal of the American Academy of Child and Adolescent Psychiatry*, **43**, 686–698.

Ratey, J., Sovner, R., Parks, J., *et al* (1991) Buspirone treatment of aggression and anxiety in mentally retarded patients: a multiple-baseline, placebo lead-in study. *Journal of Clinical Psychiatry*, **52**, 159–162.

Shea, S., Turgay, A., Carroll, A., *et al* (2004) Risperidone in the treatment of disruptive behavioral symptoms in children with autistic and other pervasive developmental disorders. *Pediatrics*, **114**, e631–e641.

Turk, J. (2003) Melatonin supplementation for severe and intractable sleep disturbance in young people with developmental disabilities: short review and commentary. *Journal of Medical Genetics*, **40**, 793–796.

Turk, J. (2007) Drug therapy. In *Child and Adolescent Psychiatry, a Developmental Approach* (eds J. Turk, P. Graham & F. Verhulst), pp. 445–455. Oxford University Press.

Verhoeven, W. M. & Tuinier, S. (1996) The effect of buspirone on challenging behaviour in mentally retarded patients: an open prospective multi-case study. *Journal of Intellectual Disability Research*, **40**, 502–508.

CHAPTER 9

Multi-agency working

Which agencies?

Depending on who is within the team, a CAMHS learning disability team will probably need close links with a number of agencies to supplement the skills mix (Table 8.1).

Liaison with tier 1

Several professionals in tier 1 (see Chapter 11) may be involved with the same families; for example specialist health visitors, special school nurses, Portage workers, child development service professionals.

All professionals should consider whether they require further training in aspects of learning disability. Are there opportunities for this be reciprocated or undertaken jointly?

At what point do different professionals involve a CAMHS learning disability service in consultation, or referral? For example, would a referral be made by a school nurse working with a family whose teenage son is showing inappropriate sexualised behaviour, or by a teacher of an autistic child who is very anxious about transitions?

Benefits

The benefits of liaison with tier 1 include:

- learning from different skills and perspectives
- complementing what the CAMHS team cannot provide
- joining up packages of care and support for families

Table 8.1 Agencies with which a CAMHS learning disability team will probably need close links

Agency	Function
Generic CAMHS	May have other disciplines to which to refer (e.g. systemic family therapy, psychotherapy, child psychiatry)
Community paediatrics	Manage medical care, especially epilepsy. May be able to organise routine blood monitoring for those patients on neuroleptic medication. May share some of the autism, ADHD assessments and management
Speech and language therapy	Contribute to assessment (particularly autistic-spectrum disorder). Contribute to interventions where supporting communication is vital
Occupational therapy	Assessment, particularly of sensory issues. May contribute to interventions that need a sensory 'diet' or physical protection (e.g. for children who self-injure)
School nurses	May already be offering general advice on feeding, sleeping, toileting, emotional and behavioural issues, sexuality, etc. May know families well and help parents to implement suggested strategies
School staff (teaching and support)	Contribute to assessment, particularly in recording behaviour in classroom setting. May know families well and help parents to implement suggested strategies
Portage	May already offer general advice on feeding, sleeping, toileting, emotional and behavioural issues, sexuality, etc. May know families well and help parents to implement the suggested strategies
Social care	Care and support packages to families. Child protection
Educational psychology	Provide information for assessments
Voluntary sector	Play and home support schemes
Adult learning disability services	May have a transition worker who will be part of the 'team around the child' planning transition

- adding variety to jobs, in terms of both colleagues and settings
- feeling valued by other agencies.

Difficulties

- *Different professional 'languages' and 'cultures'.* For example, social care, education and child health settings may have different understandings of terms such as 'mental health problem', 'assessment', treatment'.
- *Different structures for line management.* Line management structures will determine who is able to represent the team at meetings and make decisions that have strategic or funding implications.

- *Inappropriate referrals or lack of appropriate cases referred.* Clear referral criteria are required. The use of a screening tool such as the Developmental Behaviour Checklist (Einfeld & Tonge, 1995) or ChA-PAS (Moss *et al*, 2007) or Social Communication Questionnaire (Rutter *et al*, 2003) may help to identify those with clinically significant problems.
- *Inappropriate expectations of what CAMHS can do.* The CAMHS learning disability service should draw up its own specification and communicate this to other agencies. Other agencies should be informed of its practice through training, presentations at team meetings, leaflets, and so on.
- *Different standards for sharing information and maintaining confidentiality.*
  - Is there a common understanding of Caldicott principles?
  - Is there a cross-agency agreement for information sharing already in place? If not, with whom and how could this be worked on?
  - Is there a secure system for exchanging information by email?
  - Is there a locked place for keeping written records if patients are seen in different agencies?
  - What is the policy for who can access these records, including patients and families?
  - How are records disposed of?

Virtual teams

Where the skills mix of the team is limited, it may be possible to build up a 'virtual team'. Examples might include:

- a speech and language or educational psychologist to attend a regular social communication assessment clinic
- staff from special schools co-running groups
- a social worker who agrees to be part of the 'team around the child', supporting a mother in buying toys and organising the home environment for some behavioural work in the home.

Supervision and line management structures must be clear, particularly in the work around the direct activity (e.g. writing reports, audit).

Pathways for joint working

There need to be clear, written pathways and protocols for joint working relationships. Because many of the families are struggling with the care of their children, social care services may need to provide more support. For example, support with extra respite or care in the home whilst you are working with parents to change behavioural management. Who can arrange for this Care package to be funded, resourced, recruited and reviewed? Similarly, what are the arrangements with paediatricians to undertake medical assessment or routine blood monitoring of those on neuroleptic medication?

Other relevant pathways are for demarcating the referral routes between tiers 1 and 2/3 and between child and adult services. The protocols need to cover a range of operational standards, including sharing information and confidentiality, documentation of clinical reports and correspondence, monitoring of clinical activity and effectiveness.

Consultation

There are many issues surrounding consultation. Teams will have to decide:

- whether consultation is given on general themes or the specific problems of particular cases
- whether they consult on an 'issue' rather than a 'named-patient' basis and whether the appropriate consent from parents or carers is required
- whether consultation is used to discuss referrals or to provide clinical advice
- how the consultation is documented and where records are kept
- who is clinically responsible for the advice given.

Strategy

Professionals working with different agencies will be asked to attend a large number of meetings. They may need to prioritise and find ways to keep up to date with the meetings they cannot attend. They need to work out how their team is represented at a local strategic level.

Further reading

Einfeld, S. L. & Tonge, B. J. (1995) The Developmental Behaviour Checklist: the development and validation of an instrument to assess behavioural and emotional disturbance in children and adolescents with mental retardation. *Journal of Autism & Developmental Disorders*, **25**, 81–104.

Miller, A., Gulliford, A. & Slringer, P. (2006) *Psychological Perspectives in Multi-agency Working (Educational & Child Psychology)*. British Psychological Society

Moss, S., Friedlander, R. & Lee, A. (2007) *The ChA-PAS Interview: The Child and Adolescent Psychiatric Assessment Schedule (ChA-PAS)*. Pavilion.

Rutter, M., Bailey, A. & Lord, C. (2003) *Social Communication Questionnaire*. GL Assessment.

Turk, J., Graham, P. & Verhulst, T. (2007) Services. In *Child & Adolescent Psychiatry: A Developmental Approach*, pp. 459–488. Oxford University Press.

CHAPTER 10

Working in partnership with families

Most children and young people with learning disabilities live with their families at home. Although it is very obvious, it is important to remember that a child cannot be considered in isolation – he or she is a son, daughter, brother, sister, grandchild, cousin, niece or nephew.

Diversity

- Family situations vary enormously.
- None the less, the same 'general life issues' (bereavement, illness, etc.) happen to these families as they do to everyone else, in addition to the complexities of supporting a child with a disability.

Expertise

- Families provide the vast majority of care and support for their child.
- Families will vary in their knowledge and understanding of the nature of their child's disability, *but*:
  - Families know their child very well and are a valuable source of information.
  - Families are important advocates for their child with a learning disability.
  - Families may provide a high level of very specialised care and support for their child with little support themselves and minimal respite.
- Families want to feel listened to yet often report feeling they do not receive this courtesy.

Effective support

- Families require information to be provided in an accessible manner (according to individual need and circumstances).

- Families do not care how the support they receive is funded or organised – they just want to access the support their child requires for a good quality of life.
- Families need support that is practical, timely and tailored to individual need.
- This covers all aspects of support, from appointments with professionals to intervention programmes.
- Any treatment for the child should take into account the effect on the family.
- The complex systems and processes that are in place to support families are often fragmented and difficult to negotiate. Every effort should be made by professionals to provide a range of seamless and coordinated supports to the family.
- Families and professionals should all be working towards the same shared goals. Most goals can be achieved when professionals work as equal partners with families. This means the professionals should listen to the families, value their knowledge and experience, and understand what things are important for them.

CHAPTER 11

Service tiers and models

There are four tiers of service:

1 primary – front-line clinical services
2 secondary – unidisciplinary specialist services, often community based
3 tertiary – multidisciplinary specialist services
4 quarternary – highly specialised/super-regional services.

Mental health provision for children and young people with learning disability should, where possible, be embedded within generic, local CAMHS, that is, as part of existing CAMHS provision, with allocation dependent on age, needs, locality, degree of learning disability. Such a service requires:

- ring-fencing of professional time
- identification of 'champions'
- commitment from all to become involved
- collaborations with colleagues in child health, education, social services and the private and voluntary sectors.

In certain instances, highly specialist CAMHS learning disability services may exist. Life-span services for individuals with learning disability who have mental health problems may have historically served this client group, and may continue to provide a high-quality, progressive service, or other agencies such as community and developmental paediatrics or clinical psychology may act as local champions. However, there are national and international legal as well as clinical imperatives dictating that children and young people with mental health problems must be helped by child and adolescent mental health services irrespective of the nature, number and severity of their disabilities.

Index

Compiled by Caroline Sheard